The Comprehensive Anti-inflammatory Diet Cookbook

Explore the World of Anti-Inflammatory Food in 25 Recipes

BY: SOPHIA FREEMAN

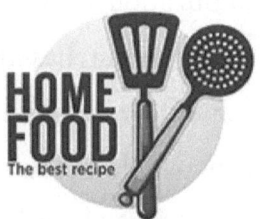

Liability

This publication is meant as an informational tool. The individual purchaser accepts all liability if damages occur because of following the directions or guidelines set out in this publication. The Author bears no responsibility for reparations caused by the misuse or misinterpretation of the content.

Copyright

The content of this publication is solely for entertainment purposes and is meant to be purchased by one individual. Permission is not given to any individual who copies, sells or distributes parts or the whole of this publication unless it is explicitly given by the Author in writing.

My gift to you!

Thank you, cherished reader, for purchasing my book and taking the time to read it. As a special reward for your decision, I would like to offer a gift of free and discounted books directly to your inbox. All you need to do is fill in the box below with your email address and name to start getting amazing offers in the comfort of your own home. You will never miss an offer because a reminder will be sent to you. Never miss a deal and get great deals without having to leave the house! Subscribe now and start saving!

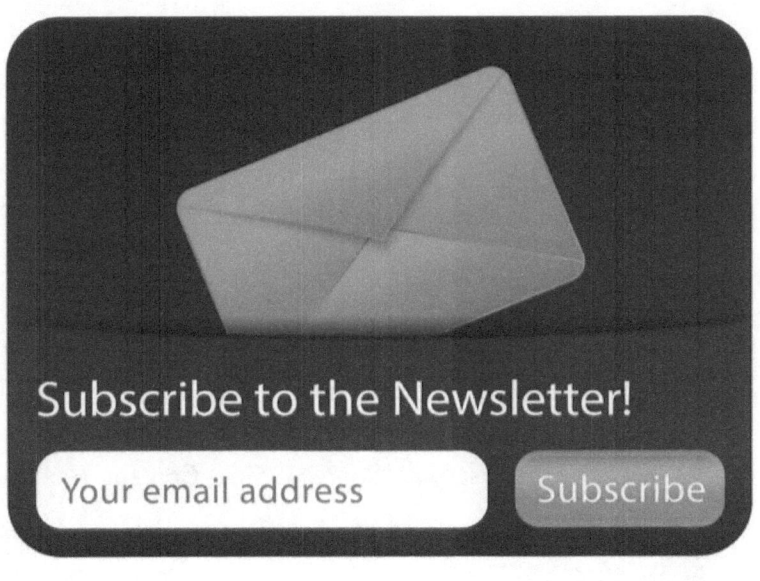

Subscribe to the Newsletter!

Your email address | Subscribe

Table of Contents

Top 10 Rules of The Anti-Inflammatory Diet

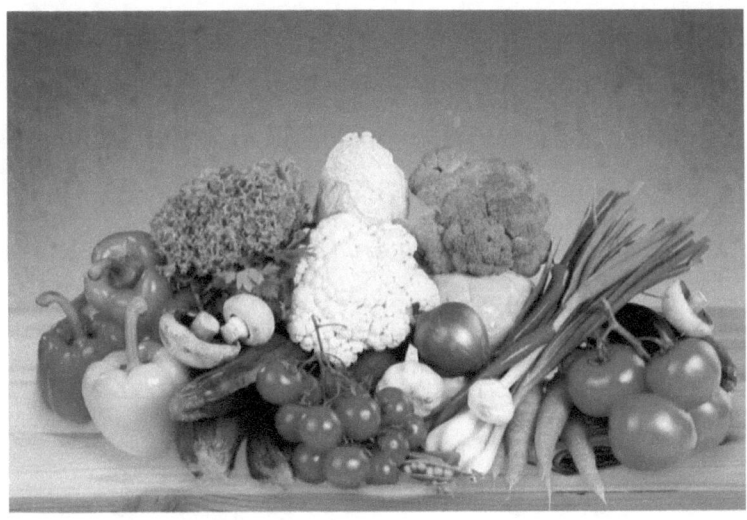

By following the anti-inflammatory diet one can easily cut down on the amount of inflammation currently plaguing their body as well as help to live a much healthier lifestyle. But the questions are, how does one follow the anti-inflammatory diet correctly without putting their body more at risk? In this section you will learn about the top 10 rules of the anti-inflammatory diet so you can help ensure you are following it correctly.

zzzzzzzzzzzzzzzzzzzzzzzzzzzzzzzzzzzzzzzzzzzzzzzzzzz

1) Make Sure That You Eat a Minimum of 9 Servings of Fruits and Veggies Every Single Day

You need to keep in mind that when you eat a serving of fruits or veggies a day, it is considered to be at least a half a cup, either cooked or raw. That is why is important when following the anti-inflammatory diet that you eat at least 9 servings of both fruits and veggies every single day.

zzzzzzzzzzzzzzzzzzzzzzzzzzzzzzzzzzzzzzzzzzzzzzzzz

2) Make Sure That You Consume at Least 25 Grams of Fiber Every Day

A diet that is rich in fiber does not only help reduce the amount of inflammation that is occurring in your body, but it also does this by helping to supply your body with naturally occurring anti-inflammatory properties that are easily found in the various fruits, vegetables and other foods.

In order to ensure that you are eating the highest amount of fiber throughout the day possible I highly recommend that you seek out foods that contain a lot of fiber such as okra, eggplant, bananas, and blueberries.

ZZZZZZZZZZZZZZZZZZZZZZZZZZZZZZZZZZZZZZZZZZZZZZZZZ

3) Limit How Much Saturated Fat You Consume on a Daily Basis

In order to reduce the amount of inflammation that you have currently occurring in your body you want to limit the amount of saturated fats that you consume on a daily basis to as much as 10% only per day. This means making sure that you limit the amount of red meat you consume on a daily basis as well as what kind of herbs and spices you are using to marinate your meat.

zzzzzzzzzzzzzzzzzzzzzzzzzzzzzzzzzzzzzzzzzzzzzzzz

4) Make Sure to Consume 4 Servings of Crucifers and Alliums

In order to ensure that you are following the anti-inflammatory diet correctly, you want to make sure that you consume both alliums and crucifers every single day. The reason why you want to include this in your diet is because they are packed full of powerful antioxidants which can help reduce the amount of inflammation occurring in your body as well as lower the risk of cancer in your body. Consume foods that are high in these properties such as broccoli, collard greens, Brussel sprouts, and cabbage.

zzzzzzzzzzzzzzzzzzzzzzzzzzzzzzzzzzzzzzzzzzzzzzzzzzz

5) Consume Fish at Least 3 Times Per Week

Even though you are cutting back on the amount of meat you are consuming on a daily basis that does not mean that you cannot eat some type of meat as a way to gain protein. With the anti-inflammatory diet you will be consuming fish at least 3 times a week. Fish contains healthy levels of healthy fats as well as omega-3 acids which you need in order to reduce the amount of inflammation in your body.

zzzzzzzzzzzzzzzzzzzzzzzzzzzzzzzzzzzzzzzzzzzzzzzz

6) Consume Foods That Are Rich in Omega 3 Fatty Acids

There have been numerous studies conducted that have found when you consume omega-3 fatty acids on a daily basis not only can It help reduce the amount of inflammation that is occurring in your body, but it can also help reduce the risk of cardiac diseases from occurring such as heart disease or cancer. What is more is that most of these conditions often have a very high inflammatory process as the root of their cause.

That is why is important to consume foods high in omega-3 fatty acids such as walnuts and various beans.

zzzzzzzzzzzzzzzzzzzzzzzzzzzzzzzzzzzzzzzzzzzzzzzz

7) Consume at Least 2 Healthy Snacks a Day

If you are the type of person that needs to snack on something at least one to two times a day, then make sure that you do just that. However, make sure that you snack on at least two healthy snacks a day instead of junk food. This means enjoying snacks such as Greek yogurt, nuts, celery sticks, walnuts, or carrots.

zzzzzzzzzzzzzzzzzzzzzzzzzzzzzzzzzzzzzzzzzzzzzzzzzzz

8) Make Sure to Use Fat Sources That Contain Healthy Properties

In order to survive your body needs fat. That fact is not hidden from anybody. However, the type of fat that you use can have an effect on your body. This is why with the anti-inflammatory diet you need to make sure that you are using fat sources that are considered to be healthy at such as sunflower oil or safflower oil.

zzzzzzzzzzzzzzzzzzzzzzzzzzzzzzzzzzzzzzzzzzzzzzzzzzz

9) Cut Out Trans Fats Completely

A good rule of thumb to follow when following the anti-inflammatory diet is to make sure that you read the labels carefully of your food. This means making sure that when you read the label you avoid foods that contain any trans fats or contain words such as hydrogenated oils.

ZZZZZZZZZZZZZZZZZZZZZZZZZZZZZZZZZZZZZZZZZZZZZZZZ

10) Avoid Any Food with Processed Sugars

It goes without saying that in order to follow the anti-inflammatory diet properly you need to make sure that you do not consume food that contains refined sugars or are processed. There are various dangers associated with these types of foods but most strikingly they are known for causing inflammation in your body and can even make the inflammation in your body worse.

zzzzzzzzzzzzzzzzzzzzzzzzzzzzzzzzzzzzzzzzzzzzzzzzzz

Anti-inflammatory Diet Recipes

zzzzzzzzzzzzzzzzzzzzzzzzzzzzzzzzzzzzzzzzzzzzzzzzzz

1) Healthy Salmon and Quinoa Bowls

This is a filling, healthy and absolutely delicious dish that you are going to want to make over and over again. Feel free to bring this dish with you to work and have all of your co-workers look at your dish with envy.

Serving Sizes: 4 Servings

Preparation Time: 30 Minutes

Ingredient List:

- 1 Cup of Quinoa, White in Color
- 1 Bunch of Kale, Your Favorite Kind
- 1 Carrot, Medium in Size, Peeled and Sliced Thinly
- 2 Tablespoons of Lemon Juice, Fresh
- 2 Cloves of Garlic, Minced
- Some Olive Oil, Extra Virgin Variety
- Dash of Sea Salt, For Taste
- 2 Cups of Chickpeas, Rinsed and Drained
- ¼ Cup of Currants, Dried
- 1 tablespoon of Hemp Seeds, Optional
- 4 Salmon Fillets

Ingredients for Your Sauce:

- ¼ Cup of Tahini Paste
- ½ Cup of Water, Warm
- 1 tablespoon of Lemon Juice, Fresh
- ½ Cup of Yogurt, Greek Variety
- ½ teaspoons of Sea Salt, For Taste

zzzzzzzzzzzzzzzzzzzzzzzzzzzzzzzzzzzzzzzzzzzzzzzzz

Instructions:

1. Use a medium sized saucepan and combine your water with your quinoa. Bring this mixture to a boil and reduce the heat to low. Cook for at least 15 minutes or until the water has disappeared and your quinoa is tender to the touch. Remove from heat and whisk with a fork to make it fluffy. Set aside for later use.

2. While your quinoa is cooking use a large sized mixing bowl and mix together your next 6 ingredients until thoroughly combined.

3. Then add in your cooked quinoa along with your next 3 ingredients. Mix well to combine and season however you wish.

4. Next heat up some oil in a large sized skillet. While your skillet is heating up dry your salmon with a paper towel and season with some salt. Once your skillet is hot enough add in your salmon with the skin side down and cook over high heat until nicely browned on all sides. This should take 2 to 3 minutes.

5. Divide your quinoa and top off with your seared salmon.

6. Next using medium sized mixing bowl and whisk together all of the ingredients for your sauce until smooth in consistency. Spoon over your fish and quinoa and serve immediately.

2) Healthy Black Bean and Sweet Potato Burgers

If you are looking for a vegetarian and vegan style dish to enjoy, then this is the perfect meal for you. Feel free to top this burger with whatever toppings you wish.

Serving Sizes: 6 Servings

Preparation Time: 1 Hour and 5 Minutes

Ingredient List:

- ½ Cup of Quinoa
- 1, 10 Ounce Can of Black Beans, rinsed and Drained
- 1 Sweet Potato, Large in Size
- ½ Cup of Red Onion, Finely Diced
- 2 Cloves of Garlic, Minced
- ½ Cup of Cilantro, Fresh and Roughly Chopped
- ½ of a Jalapeno, Seeded and Finely Diced
- 1 teaspoon of Cumin, Ground
- 2 teaspoons of Cajun Seasoning, Spicy Variety
- ¼ cup of Flour, Oat and Gluten Free
- Dash of Salt and Pepper, For Taste
- Some Oil, Coconut Variety and for Cooking
- 6 Hamburger Buns, Whole Grain Variety

Ingredients for Your Avocado and Cilantro Crema:

- ½ of an Avocado, Large in Size, Ripe and Finely Diced
- ¼ Cup of Sour Cream, Low Fat Variety
- 2 Tablespoons of Cilantro, Roughly Chopped
- 1 teaspoon of Lime Juice, Fresh
- Dash of Hot Sauce, Your Favorite Kind
- Dash of Salt, For Taste

zzz

Instructions:

1. The first thing that you want to do is cook your quinoa. To do this rinse your quinoa with some cold water until the water begins to run clear. Then add to a medium sized saucepan along with 1 cup of water. Heat over medium heat and bring to a boil. Add in your quinoa and reduce the heat to low. Allow to simmer for the next 15 minutes or until all of the water has been absorbed. Remove from heat and fluff with a fork. Set aside to cool.

2. Next poke a few holes in your sweet potato with a fork and place into your microwave to cook for the next 3 to 4 minutes or until soft to the touch.

3. Then use a food processor and add in your cooked sweet potato, beans, and next 6 ingredients. Pulse until smooth in consistency and season with a touch of salt and pepper. Pour into a bowl.

4. Add in your oat bran / oat flour and shape your mixture into 6 sized patties. Place your patties onto a baking sheet lined with some parchment paper and place into your fridge to chill for 30 minutes.

5. Next make your avocado cilantro crema. To do this use a food processor and add in all of your ingredients for your creamer. Blend on the highest setting until smooth in consistency and season with some salt.

6. After this time heat up a large sized skillet over medium to high heat. Spray with some cooking spray and place your patties onto it once it is hot enough. Cook for at least 3 to 4 minutes on each side or until golden brown in color. Remove and serve with your ready-made crema and desired toppings. Enjoy.

3) Kale Style Cesar Salad and Chicken Wrap

Here is another healthy and delicious lunch or dinner dish you are going to want to make over and over again. It is incredibly filling with low calories so you don't have to feel guilty about enjoying it.

Serving Sizes: 2 Servings

Preparation Time: 20 Minutes

Ingredient List:

- 8 Ounces of Chicken, Grilled and Thinly Sliced
- 6 Cups of Kale, Curly Variety and Cut into Small Sized Pieces
- 1 Cup of Tomatoes, Cherry Variety and Cut into Quarters
- ¾ Cup of Parmesan Cheese, Finely Shredded
- ½ and Egg, Coddles Variety and Fully Cooked
- 1 Clove of Garlic, Minced
- ½ teaspoons of Mustard, Dijon Variety
- 1 teaspoon of Honey, Raw
- 1/8 Cup of Lemon Juice, Fresh
- 1/8 Cup of Olive Oil, Extra Virgin Variety
- Dash of Salt and Pepper, For Taste
- 2 Tortillas, Whole Grain Variety and Large in Size

zzzzzzzzzzzzzzzzzzzzzzzzzzzzzzzzzzzzzzzzzzzzzzzzzz

Instructions:

1. Using a large sized bowl mix together your egg, garlic, honey, fresh lemon juice, touch of olive oil, and mustard until thoroughly mixed. Season with some salt and pepper and whisk. Set aside for later use.

2. Next add in your remaining ingredients except for your wraps into a large sized salad bowl and toss thoroughly to combine.

3. Evenly scoop out some of your salad onto your wraps and top off with some Parmesan cheese. Roll up burrito style and serve with your dressing immediately. Enjoy.

4) Cherry and Coconut Porridge

This is the perfect dish for you to make if you want a healthy yet nutritious breakfast meal that you can enjoy any day that you wish. It is easy to make and can easily be made to take along on the road with you.

Serving Sizes: 2 Servings

Preparation Time: 20 Minutes

Ingredient List:

- 1 ½ Cups of Oats, Your Favorite Kind
- 4 Tablespoons of Chia Seeds
- 3 to 4 Cups of Milk, Coconut Variety
- 3 Tablespoons of Cacao, Raw Variety
- Dash of Stevia
- Some Coconut, Shavings Only and for Topping
- 5 Cherries, Fresh Preferable
- Some Chocolate, Shavings Only and for topping
- Maple Syrup, For Topping

zzzzzzzzzzzzzzzzzzzzzzzzzzzzzzzzzzzzzzzzzzzzzzzzzzz

Instructions:

1. The first thing that you will want to do is mix together your first 5 ingredients in a large sized saucepan and place over medium heat. Bring this mixture to a boil.

2. Reduce the heat to low and allow to simmer for the next 15 minutes or until your oats are completely cooked through.

3. Pour your oatmeal into a serving bowl and top with your remaining ingredients. Serve while still piping hot and enjoy.

5) Healthy Red Quinoa Salad with Greens

This healthy quinoa recipe is packed full of roasted carrots and parsnips, making this a dish you will want to enjoy if you wish to live a healthier lifestyle. For the tastiest results feel free to serve this dish with your favorite kind of salad dressing.

Serving Sizes: 4 Servings

Preparation Time: 35 Minutes

Ingredient List:

- 1 Onion, Yellow in Color, Small in Size and Thinly Sliced
- 2 Carrots, Medium in Size, Peeled and Cut into Small Sized Pieces
- 2 Parsnips, Medium in Size, Peeled and Cut into Small Sized Pieces
- 1 tablespoon of Olive Oil, Extra Virgin Variety
- ½ teaspoons of Sea Salt, For Taste
- 4 Sprigs of Thyme, Fresh
- 1 Cup of Quinoa, Red in Color

zzzzzzzzzzzzzzzzzzzzzzzzzzzzzzzzzzzzzzzzzzzzzzzzz

Instructions:

1. First preheat your oven to 425 degrees.

2. Next use a large sized bowl and toss your first five ingredients together until thoroughly coated.

3. Place this mixture onto your baking sheet lined with parchment paper in a single layer and top off with your fresh thyme.

4. Place into your oven to bake for the next 30 minutes or until golden brown and caramelized.

5. While your mixture is baking cook up your quinoa. To do this bring your quinoa and water together in a medium sized saucepan. Cook for at least 15 minutes over low heat or until all of the liquid has been absorbed and your quinoa is tender to the touch. Season with some salt and pepper and set aside.

6. Add in your roasted vegetables to your quinoa and thoroughly to combine.

7. Transfer to a serving dish and drizzle with your favorite salad dressing. Enjoy.

6) Poached Eggs and Curried Potatoes

This is a great tasting recipe to make if you are looking for a light and hearty meal. It has just the perfect touch of spice, making it perfect for those who are craving some spicy food.

Serving Sizes: 4 Servings

Preparation Time: 40 Minutes

Ingredient List:

- 2 Potatoes, Russet Variety
- 1 Piece of Ginger, Fresh, Peeled and minced
- 2 Cloves of Garlic, Minced
- 1 tablespoon of Olive Oil, Extra Virgin Variety
- 2 Tablespoons of Curry, Powdered Variety
- 1, 15 Ounce Can of Tomato Sauce
- 4 Eggs, Large in Size
- ½ Bunch of Cilantro, Fresh and Roughly Chopped

zzzzzzzzzzzzzzzzzzzzzzzzzzzzzzzzzzzzzzzzzzzzzzzzzzz

Instructions:

1. The first thing that you will want to do is wash your potatoes thoroughly. Then cut them into small sized cubes. Place into a pot of water and bring to a boil over medium heat. Boil for the next 5 to 6 minutes or until your potatoes are tender to the touch. Drain and set aside.

2. While your potatoes are boiling, make your sauce. To do this add your next 2 ingredients in a large sized saucepan placed over medium heat. Cook for the next 2 minutes or until soft to the touch.

3. Then add in your curry powder and stir thoroughly to combine.

4. Add in your tomato sauce and stir again to combine. Taste your sauce and add in some salt for taste if you desire.

5. Toss in your cooked potatoes and stir thoroughly until evenly mixed. Add in water to your mixture if it is too dry.

6. Make 4 even sized wells in your potato mixture and crack your eggs into them. Continue to cook for the next 6 to 10 minutes or until your eggs are fully set.

7. Remove from heat and garnish with your cilantro. Enjoy whenever you are ready.

7) Honey Roasted Carrots

Here is a delicious and healthy recipe I know you will not be able to get enough of. For the tastiest results I highly recommend that you only use the freshest carrots possible.

Serving Sizes: 4 Servings

Preparation Time: 35 Minutes

Ingredient List:

- 1 Bunch of Carrots, Large in Size and Scrubbed
- 2 Tablespoons of Olive Oil, Extra Virgin Variety
- 1 tablespoon of Honey, Raw
- ½ teaspoons of Sea Salt, For Taste
- ½ teaspoons of Thyme, Dried

zzzzzzzzzzzzzzzzzzzzzzzzzzzzzzzzzzzzzzzzzzzzzzzzzzz

Instructions:

1. First preheat your oven to 425 degrees. While your oven is heating up line a baking sheet with some parchment paper.

2. Next toss your carrots with your oil and next 3 ingredients until thoroughly coated.

3. Place this mixture into an even layer on your baking sheet.

4. Place into your oven to bake for the next 30 minutes or until brown and caramelized.

5. Remove and allow to cool completely. Serve whenever you are ready.

8) Healthy Raspberry and Avocado Smoothie

While this smoothie may contain a few ingredients that may not seem as if they pair well together, once you get a taste of it yourself I know you are going to love it. It is packed full of important vitamins and nutrients, making it one of the bets anti-inflammatory recipes I know you will love.

Serving Sizes: 1 Servings

Preparation Time: 5 Minutes

Ingredient List:

- 1 Avocado, Peeled and Pitted
- ¾ Cup of Orange Juice, Fresh
- ¾ Cup of Raspberry Juice, Fresh
- ½ Cup of Raspberries Fresh

ZZZZZZZZZZZZZZZZZZZZZZZZZZZZZZZZZZZZZZZZZZZZZZZZZZZZ

Instructions:

1. Place all of your ingredients into a blender.

2. Blend on the highest setting until smooth in consistency.

3. Pour your mixture into a chilled glass and serve right away. Enjoy.

9) Coconut Style Kale Salad with Avocado

Here is a healthy kale salad recipe that I know you are going to fall in love with. This is a great salad to enjoy whenever you want to detox your body or whenever you are looking for something a little healthy to enjoy.

Serving Sizes: 4 Servings

Preparation Time: 25 Minutes

Ingredient List:

- 1 Bunch of Kale, Your Favorite Kind
- 1 Clove of Garlic, Minced
- 2 Tablespoons of Lemon Juice, Fresh
- 2 Tablespoons of Aminos, Liquid Variety
- 1 tablespoon of Olive Oil, Extra Virgin Variety
- 2 Tablespoons of Oil, Coconut Variety, Organic, Extra Virgin Variety and Melted
- 6 Radishes, Thinly Sliced
- 2 Carrots, Medium in Size and Sliced Thinly
- 2 Tablespoons of Vinegar, Apple Cider Variety
- 1 teaspoon of Sea Salt, For Taste
- 1/3 Cup of Coconut, Flaked
- 1 Avocado, Finely Diced

zzzzzzzzzzzzzzzzzzzzzzzzzzzzzzzzzzzzzzzzzzzzzzzzz

Instructions:

1. The first thing that you want to do is remove the ribs from your kale and then stick your kale on top of one another in a pile. Roll up similar to a cigar and thinly slice it. Place into a large sized mixing bowl.

2. Then add in your next 4 ingredients and stir to combine.

3. Drizzle in your coconut oil and stir thoroughly to coat. Set this aside for the next 15 minutes, making sure to stir once in a while or until everything begins to wilt.

4. Using a small sized bowl mix together your next 4 ingredients and allow to sit for the next 15 minutes until your vegetables are tender to the touch.

5. Meanwhile toast your coconut in a large sized skillet placed over medium heat until golden brown in color. This should take at least two minutes. Remove and set aside for later use.

6. Add your pickled veggies to your kale salad along with your avocado. Toss thoroughly to combine and serve with a garnish of your coconut. Enjoy.

10) Mediterranean Style Tuna Salad

Here is a salad recipe that I know you are going to love. It is light and hearty, making it perfect when you don't want something too filling. For the tastiest results I highly recommend serving this dish between two slices of your favorite kind of bread.

Serving Sizes: 2 Servings

Preparation Time: 5 Minutes

Ingredient List:

- 2, 5 Ounce Cans of Tuna, packed in Water and Drained
- ¼ Cup of Mayonnaise, Your Favorite Kind
- ¼ Cup of Kalamata, Finely Chopped
- 2 Tablespoons of Red Onion, Minced
- 2 Tablespoons of Red Peppers, Fire Roasted and Finely Chopped
- 2 Tablespoons of Basil, Fresh and Roughly Chopped
- 1 tablespoon of Capers
- 1 tablespoon of Lemon Juice, Fresh
- Dash of Salt and Pepper, For Taste
- 2 Tomatoes, Large in Size and Vine Ripened Variety

zzzzzzzzzzzzzzzzzzzzzzzzzzzzzzzzzzzzzzzzzzzzzzzzzz

Instructions:

1. First add all of your ingredients except for your tomatoes into a large sized bowl. Stir thoroughly to combine.

2. Thinly slice your tomatoes into sixths, making sure that you do not cut them all the way through. Gently pry your tomatoes open and scoop as much of your salad mixture into the center.

3. Serve Immediately and enjoy.

11) Moroccan Style Red Lentil Soup

Here is yet another delicious soup recipe that I know for sure you won't be able to get enough of. Make this when you are feeling a bit under the weather to give you the pick-me-up that you desperately need.

Serving Sizes: 4 Servings

Preparation Time: 35 Minutes

Ingredient List:

- 2 Tablespoons of Olive Oil, Extra Virgin Variety
- 1 Onion, Medium in Size, Yellow in Color and Finely Diced
- 2 Carrots, Medium in Size and Finely Diced
- 2 Cloves of Garlic, Minced
- 1 teaspoon of Cumin, Ground Variety
- ½ teaspoons of Ginger, Ground Variety
- ½ teaspoons of Turmeric, Ground Variety
- ½ teaspoons of Red Chili Flakes
- ½ teaspoons of Sea Salt, For Taste
- 1, 15 Ounce Can of Tomatoes, Finely Diced
- 1 Cup of Red Lentils, Dried and Split
- 2 Quarts of Stock, Vegetable Variety
- 1 Bunch of Chards, Stems Removed and Chopped Roughly

zzzzzzzzzzzzzzzzzzzzzzzzzzzzzzzzzzzzzzzzzzzzzzzzz

Instructions:

1. Use a large sized stock pot set over medium heat. Add in your oil and once your oil is hot enough add in your onions and carrots. Cook until soft to the touch. This should take at least 7 minutes.

2. Then add in your next 6 ingredients and stir thoroughly took combined. Cook for an additional minute.

3. Add in your tomatoes and continue to cook until your tomatoes are soft to the touch. This should take at least five minutes.

4. Next add in your stock and your lentils and bring your mixture to a boil. Once your mixture is boiling reduce the heat to low and then allow to simmer for the next 10 minutes or until your lentils are soft to the touch.

5. Gently fold in your chard and continue to cook until slightly wilted. Remove from heat.

6. Serve with a wedge of lemon and a dollop of Greek yogurt and enjoy.

12) Slow Cooker Style Turkey Chili

If you are a huge fan of chili, then this is one recipe that I know you are going to fall in love with. Incredibly easy to make and absolutely filling, I know you won't be able to get enough of it.

Serving Sizes: 8 to 10 Servings

Preparation Time: 4 to 6 Hours

Ingredient List:

- 1 tablespoon of Olive Oil, Extra Virgin Variety
- 1 Pound of Turkey, Lean and Ground
- 1 Onion, Medium in Size and Finely Diced
- 1 Red Pepper, Finely Chopped
- 1 Yellow Pepper, Finely Chopped
- 2, 15 Ounce Cans of Tomato Sauce
- 2, 15 Ounce Cans of Tomatoes, Petite Variety and Finely Diced
- 2, 15 Ounce Cans of Black Beans, Rinsed and Drained
- 2, 15 Ounce Cans of Kidney Beans, Rinsed and Drained
- 1, 16 Ounce Jar of Jalapeno Peppers, Deli-Sliced Variety and Drained
- 1 Cup of Corn, Frozen Variety
- 2 Tablespoons of Chili, Powdered Variety
- 1 tablespoon of Cumin, Ground Variety
- Dash of Salt and Pepper, For Taste
- Some Green Onions, Finely Chopped and for Topping
- Some Cheese, Shredded and for Topping
- Some Sour Cream, For Topping
- Some Avocado, For Topping

zzz

Instructions:

1. The first thing you want to do is heat up some oil in a large sized skillet place over medium heat. Once the oil is hot enough add in your turkey and cook until brown in color.

2. Once your turkey is brown transfer it to your slow cooker.

3. Then add in your remaining ingredients and stir thoroughly to combine.

4. Cover and cook on the highest setting for the next 4 hours or on the lowest setting for the next 6 hours.

5. After this time serve with your desired toppings and enjoy.

13) Black Fried Rice Smothered in Peas and Scallions

Here is a light and filling dish that you can make whenever you are craving it. Make this dish to accompany your main meal or serve it alone as it is. Either way I know you are going to love it.

Serving Sizes: 4 Servings

Preparation Time: 20 Minutes

Ingredient List:

- 2 Tablespoons of Oil, Coconut Variety, Organic and Extra Virgin Variety
- 2 Carrots, Medium in Size and Finely Diced
- 1 Onion, Yellow in Color, Small in Size and Finely Diced
- 1 Bunch of Scallions, Parts Separated and Thinly Sliced
- 1 Cup of Snap Peas, Thinly Sliced
- 2 Cloves of Garlic, Minced
- 1 tablespoon of Ginger, Fresh and Minced
- 3 Cups of Black Rice, Fully Cooked
- 2 Tablespoons of Aminos, Liquid Variety
- 2 teaspoons of Oil, Sesame Variety and Lightly Toasted
- 1 teaspoon of Sriracha
- 2 Eggs, Large in Size and Beaten Lightly
- 1 tablespoon of Hemp Seed, Organic Variety and Shelled

ZZZZZZZZZZZZZZZZZZZZZZZZZZZZZZZZZZZZZZZZZZZZZZZZ

Instructions:

1. Use a large sized wok and heat up your coconut oil. Once the coconut oil is hot enough add in your next three ingredients and cook over high heat until soft to the touch. This should take at least five minutes.

2. Then add in your next 4 ingredients and cook for the next 2 minutes.

3. Gently fold in your rice and continue cooking until thoroughly coated.

4. Add in your next 3 ingredients and stir thoroughly to combine.

5. Make a well in your rice mixture and pour in your eggs directly into the center, making sure to stir gently. Cook until nearly set.

6. Toss your mixture with your hemp seed and remove from heat. Serve while still piping hot and enjoy.

14) Gingerbread Style Oatmeal

Here is another oatmeal recipe that I know you won't be able to get enough of. It is a filling breakfast dish that you can make when you find yourself too tight on time and need something quick to make.

Serving Sizes: 4 Servings

Preparation Time: 20 Minutes

Ingredient List:

- 4 Cups of Water, Warm
- 1 Cup of Oats, Steel Cut Variety
- 1 ½ Tablespoons of Cinnamon, Ground Variety
- ¼ teaspoons of Coriander, Ground Variety
- 1 teaspoon of Cloves, Ground Variety
- ¼ teaspoons of Ginger, Ground Variety
- ¼ teaspoons of Allspice, Ground Variety
- 1/8 teaspoons of Nutmeg, Ground Variety
- ¼ teaspoons of Cardamom, Ground Variety
- Some Maple Syrup, For Serving and Your Favorite Kind

ZZ

Instructions:

1. The first thing that you will want to do is cook your oats according to the directions on the package. When you are cooking them include your spices and water as well.

2. Once finished cooking add in some maple syrup and serve whenever you are ready.

15) Sesame Style Shrimp Stir Fry

If you are craving Asian cuisine, then this is the perfect dish for you to make. Feel free to top this dish with whatever toppings you wish to make this dish truly unique.

Serving Sizes: 4 Servings

Preparation Time: 20 Minutes

Ingredient List:

- ¼ Cup of Aminos, Liquid Variety
- 2 teaspoons of Oil, Sesame Variety
- 2 Tablespoons of Honey, Raw
- 2 Tablespoons of Hemp Seed, Organic and Shelled
- 2 Tablespoons of Oil, Coconut Variety, Extra Virgin Variety and Evenly Divided
- 1 Pound of Shrimp, Peeled and Deveined
- 1 Onion, Yellow in Color, Small in Size and Sliced Thinly
- 1 Bell Pepper, Red or Orange in Color, Seeded and Sliced Thinly
- 1 Yellow Squash, Small in Size and Cut into Small Piece
- 3 Ounces of Mushrooms, Shitake Variety, Stems Removed and Thinly Sliced
- 2 Cloves of Garlic, Minced
- 2 Cups of Chard, Rainbow Variety and Thinly Sliced

zzzzzzzzzzzzzzzzzzzzzzzzzzzzzzzzzzzzzzzzzzzzzzzzzz

Instructions:

1. First use a small sized mixing bowl and whisk together your first three ingredients until thoroughly combined.

2. Then use a large sized wok and heat up your coconut oil over medium heat. Once your oil is hot enough add in your shrimp and cook for the next 2 minutes or until pink in color. Transfer to a bowl and set aside for later use.

3. Add in the remaining oil to your work and stir fry your next 4 ingredients until slightly charred. This should take about 5 minutes. Then add in your garlic and continue to cook for at least 1 minute before adding in your chard. Cook until your chard is slightly wilted.

4. Next add in your sauce and allow to simmer until thick in consistency. This take at least two minutes.

5. Remove from heat and gently fold in your shrimp until thoroughly combined. Serve while still hot and enjoy.

16) Baked Pecan and Rosemary Tilapia

This is a dish that you can make when you are looking to enjoy something on the classier side. It is perfect to make for your significant other and it is also incredibly healthy to enjoy.

Serving Sizes: 4 Servings

Preparation Time: 25 Minutes

Ingredient List:

- 1/3 Cup of Pecans, Raw and Finely Chopped
- 1/3 Cup of Breadcrumbs, Panko Variety
- 2 teaspoons of Rosemary, Fresh and Roughly Chopped
- ½ teaspoons of Brown Sugar, Light and Packed
- 1/8 teaspoons of Salt, For Taste
- Dash of Cayenne Pepper
- 1 ½ teaspoons of Olive Oil, Extra Virgin Variety
- 1 Egg, Large in Size and White Only
- 4, 4 Ounce Tilapia Fillets, Fresh

zz

Instructions:

1. The first thing that you will want to do is preheat your oven to 350 degrees.

2. Then use a small sized baking dish and stir together your first five ingredients. Stir until thoroughly combined.

3. Slowly add in your olive oil and toss to coat. Pour into your baking dish.

4. Place into your oven to bake for the next 7 to 8 minutes or until golden brown in color.

5. After this time increase the heat of your oven to 400 degrees. Spray your dish with some cooking spray.

6. Then use a small sized bowl and whisk your egg whites thoroughly.

7. Dip your tilapia into your egg white and then roll into your pecan mixture. Place your coated tilapias onto a generally greased baking dish.

8. Place into your oven to bake for the next 10 minutes or until your tilapia is fully cooked through. Remove and serve while still piping hot.

17) Hearty Quinoa and Turkey Stuffed Peppers

Here is another appetizer dish that I know you are going to fall in love with. Make this dish as an appetizer to serve to your friends and family during your next gathering.

Serving Sizes: 6 to 8 Servings

Preparation Time: 1 Hour

Ingredient List:

- 3 Peppers, Yellow in Color and Large in Size
- 1 ¼ Pound of Turkey, Lean and Ground
- 1 Cup of Tomatoes, Finely Diced
- ¼ Cup of Onion, Sweet Variety and Finely Diced
- 1 Cup of Spinach, Fresh and Roughly Chopped
- 2 teaspoons of Garlic, Minced
- 1 Cup of Tomato Sauce, Your Favorite Kind
- 1 Cup of Broth, Chicken Variety
- 1 Cup of Quinoa, Dry Variety
- Dash of Cheddar Cheese, Finely Shredded and for Topping

zz

Instructions:

1. First use a small sized saucepan and cook your quinoa according to the directions on the package. Once your quinoa is fully cooked remove from heat and set aside.

2. Then sauté your vegetables in a pan with a little bit of olive oil over medium heat.

3. Add in your ground turkey and garlic to your cooked vegetables and continue to cook until your turkey is brown in color.

4. Then add in your tomato sauce and half of your chicken broth. Allow to simmer until your turkey is fully cooked through.

5. Next preheat your oven to 400 degrees.

6. While your turkey mixture is simmering prepare your bell peppers. To do this first wash your peppers and cut them in half, making sure to remove the stems and the seats. Then spray a baking pan with a generous amount of cooking spray and place your bell peppers onto them.

7. Once your quinoa has been fully cooked add it into your pan with your turkey and vegetables and stir thoroughly to combine.

8. Stuff your peppers with this mixture until all of your mixture has been used. Top off with your cheese.

9. Place into your oven to bake for at least 30 to 35 minutes.

10. After this time remove and serve while still piping hot. Enjoy.

18) Apple, Ginger and Rhubarb Muffins

Here is a delicious muffin recipe you won't have to feel guilty about enjoying. These delicious muffins can be enjoyed any time of the day and will help to satisfy your strongest sweet tooth.

Serving Sizes: 8 Servings

Preparation Time: 35 Minutes

Ingredient List:

- ½ Cup of Meal, Almond Variety
- ¼ Cup of Sugar, Raw and Unrefined
- 2 Tablespoons of Ginger, Crystallized and Finely Chopped
- 1 tablespoon of Linseed Meal, Ground Variety
- ½ Cup of Flour, Buckwheat Variety
- ¼ Cup of Rice Flour, Fine and Brown Variety
- 2 Tablespoons of Corn flour, Organic Variety
- 2 teaspoons of Baker's Style Baking Powder, Gluten-Free Variety
- ½ teaspoons of Cinnamon, Ground Variety
- ½ teaspoons of Ginger, Ground Variety
- Dash of Sea Salt, For Taste
- 1 Cup of Rhubarb, Finely Sliced
- 1 Apple, Small in Size, Peeled, Cored and Diced Finely
- 1/3 Cup + 1 tablespoon of Milk, Rice or Almond Variety
- ¼ Cup of Olive Oil, Extra Virgin Variety
- 1 Egg, Large in Size
- 1 teaspoon of Vanilla, Pure

zzzzzzzzzzzzzzzzzzzzzzzzzzzzzzzzzzzzzzzzzzzzzzzzzz

Instructions:

1. The first thing that you will want to do is preheat your oven to 350 degrees. While your oven is heating up grease a muffin pans with some cooking spray or line with muffin cups.

2. Next mix together your first 4 ingredients into a medium sized bowl. Then add in your remaining ingredients and stir thoroughly to combine.

3. Pour your batter into your generously greased or lined muffin pan.

4. Place into your oven to bake for the next 20 to 25 minutes or until golden around the edges.

5. After this time remove from your oven and allow to cool slightly for 5 to 10 minutes before serving. Enjoy.

19) Tasty Squash and Red Lentil Stew

This is a stew recipe that you can make when you need something a little more filling. It is perfect to make on a cold winter's night or whenever you are craving some wholesome home cooking.

Serving Sizes: 4 Servings

Preparation Time: 20 Minutes

Ingredient List:

- 1 teaspoon of Olive Oil, Extra Virgin Variety
- 1 Onion, Sweet Variety and Finely Chopped
- 3 Cloves of Garlic, Minced
- 1 tablespoon of Curry, Powdered Variety
- 4 Cups of Broth, Low in Sodium and Chicken Variety
- 1 Cup of Lentils, Red in Color
- 3 Cups of Butternut Squash, Fully Cooked
- 1 Cup of Greens, Your Favorite Kind
- Dash of Ginger, Grated and for Taste
- Dash of Salt and Pepper, For Taste

zzzzzzzzzzzzzzzzzzzzzzzzzzzzzzzzzzzzzzzzzzzzzzzzzzz

Instructions:

1. First use a large sized pot and heat over medium heat. Add in your olive oil, garlic and onions and cook for at least five minutes.

2. Then add in your curry powder and continue to cook for another 5 to 10 minutes before adding in your broth and lentils.

3. Bring your mixture to a boil before reducing the heat to low and cooking for another 10 minutes.

4. Gently stir in your butternut squash and any greens that you choose to use. Continue to cook over medium heat for the next 5 to 8 minutes before removing from heat.

5. Season with some salt and pepper. Toss in your grated ginger and serve whenever you are ready.

20) Winter Style Fruit Salad

Here is yet another delicious salad recipe that you can make whenever you are looking to enjoy some sweet tasting fruit. This is perfect when all of your favorite winter fruits is in season. I know you are going to love it.

Serving Sizes: 6 Servings

Preparation Time: 5 Minutes

Ingredient List:

- 4 Persimmons, Fuya Variety and Cut into Small Sized Pieces
- 3 Pears, Bosch Variety and Cut into Small Sized Pieces
- 1 Cup of Grapes, Fresh and Cut into Halves
- ¾ Cup of Pecans, Cut into Halves

zzzzzzzzzzzzzzzzzzzzzzzzzzzzzzzzzzzzzzzzzzzzzzzzzzz

Instructions:

1. First mix together all of your ingredients for your dressing into a small size bowl until thoroughly mixed. Set aside for later use.

2. Then cut up your fruits for your salad into small sized pieces.

3. Place into a medium sized bowl and toss with your dressing until thoroughly combined.

4. Toss in your pecan pieces and serve whenever you are ready. Enjoy.

21) Gluten Free Style Crepes

Here is yet another delicious breakfast style recipe that I know you are going to fall in love with. It is easy to make and for the tastiest results I highly recommend serving this dish with your favorite fruit as a topping.

Serving Sizes: 6 Servings

Preparation Time: 15 Minutes

Ingredient List:

- 2 Eggs, Large in Size
- 1 teaspoon of Vanilla, Gluten Free Variety
- ½ Cup of Milk, Nut Variety
- ½ Cup of Water, Warm
- ¼ teaspoons of Salt, For Taste
- 1 to 2 Tablespoons of Agave Nectar
- 1 Cup of Flour, All Purpose Variety
- 2 Tablespoons of Oil, Coconut Variety and Melted
- 1 tablespoon of Oil, Coconut Variety

zzzzzzzzzzzzzzzzzzzzzzzzzzzzzzzzzzzzzzzzzzzzzzzzzzzz

Instructions:

1. First place your coconut oil into a small sized saucepan and melt over medium heat.

2. Meanwhile mix together your next 6 ingredients in a medium sized mixing bowl until thoroughly combined.

3. Slowly add in your flour and whisk thoroughly to combine.

4. After this time remove your oil from heat and pour in your batter while still whisking. Mix until smooth in consistency.

5. Then heat up some more coconut oil in a large sized frying pan placed over medium heat. Scoop at least one third cup of your batter onto your frying pan and swirl around to form the crepe.

6. Cook your crepe for at least two minutes or until the bottom of it is light brown in color. Gently flip and cook on the other side for another two minutes.

7. Repeat until all of your batter has been used up. Serve and enjoy.

22) Italian Style Stuffed Red Peppers

Here is a delicious meal that I know your family and friends are going to love. This is perfect to make when you want to make a delicious appetizer to hold your guests over until dinner is finished.

Serving Sizes: 4 Servings

Preparation Time: 40 Minutes

Ingredient List:

- 1 Pound of Turkey, Lean and Ground
- 3 Bell Peppers, Red in Color
- 2 Cups of Spaghetti Sauce, Your Favorite Kind
- 1 teaspoon of Basil and Oregano Mixed
- 1 teaspoon of Garlic, Powdered Variety
- ½ teaspoons of Salt and Pepper, For Taste
- ½ Cup of Spinach, Frozen and Roughly Chopped
- 2 Tablespoons of Parmesan Cheese, Freshly Grated

zzzzzzzzzzzzzzzzzzzzzzzzzzzzzzzzzzzzzzzzzzzzzzzzzzz

Instructions:

1. The first thing that you will want to do is preheat your oven to 450 degrees. While your oven is heating up line a large sized baking sheet with some aluminum foil.

2. Next wash and destem your red peppers. Cut them in half lengthwise and remove any seeds and ribs from the inside. Place onto your baking sheet.

3. Next cook up your turkey in a large sized skillet placed over medium to high heat until brown in color.

4. Then add in your sauce and seasonings to your pan and stir thoroughly to combine.

5. Add in your parmesan and spinach and toss until your spinach slightly wilts. Remove from heat.

6. Scoop at least half a cup of your cooked turkey mixture into each of your peppers.

7. Top off with your cheese.

8. Place into your oven to bake for the next 25 to 30 minutes or until your cheese is fully melted and golden brown in color.

9. Remove from oven and allow to cool slightly before serving.

23) Tasty Potato and Salmon Tartine

If you are looking for a delicious and creative dish to enjoy, then this is the perfect dish for you. It is easy to make and makes for a healthy and great tasting snack to enjoy whenever you want.

Serving Sizes: 4 Servings

Preparation Time: 30 Minutes

Ingredients for Your Potato Tartine:

- 1 Russet Potato, Peeled and Grated
- 2 Tablespoons of Butter, Soft
- Dash of Salt and Pepper, For Taste

Ingredients for Your Toppings:

- 4 Ounces of Goat Cheese, Soft and Warm
- 1 ½ Tablespoons of Chives, Finely Minced
- ½ of a Clove of Garlic, Minced
- ½ a Lemon, Zest Only
- Some Salmon, Smoked and Sliced Thinly
- 2 Tablespoons of Capers, Drained
- 2 Tablespoons of Red Onion, Finely Chopped
- ½ of an Egg, Hard Boiled and Finely Chopped
- Some Chives, Minced and for Garnish

zzzzzzzzzzzzzzzzzzzzzzzzzzzzzzzzzzzzzzzzzzzzzzzzzz

Instructions:

1. The first thing that you want to do is make your toppings. To do this combine your first three ingredients for your toppings into a small sized bowl. Season with a dash of salt and pepper and stir gently.

2. Gently fold in your chives and set this mixture aside.

3. Then season your red onion and hardboiled egg with a bit of salt.

Instructions to Make Potato Tartine:

1. Next grate your potatoes using the large sized holes of your grater. Then squeeze over a sink to expel the excess liquid. Season with a generous amount of salt and pepper and toss thoroughly to coat.

2. Next heat up your butter in a large sized skillet placed over medium to high heat. Once the butter is melted add in your potatoes and shape into a large sized circle. Cook for at least 8 to 10 minutes or until the bottom of your potato pancake is brown in color.

3. Carefully flip it over and continue to cook for an additional 8 to 10 minutes on the other side or until golden brown in color.

4. Remove and allow to cool on a cooling rack.

Instructions for Assembly:

1. Once your potato pancake has cooled completely spread your goat cheese mixture on top of it.

2. Next layer your salmon over it and garnish with their red onions, hard boiled eggs and capers.

3. Garnish with some chives and serve whenever you are ready.

24) Healthy Ginger and Buckwheat Granola

This is a great tasting granola recipe to make when you are looking for a quick and delicious snack to enjoy. It is light on the calories so you don't have to worry about feeling guilty about enjoying this dish.

Serving Sizes: 2 Servings

Preparation Time: 15 Minutes

Ingredient List:

- 2 Cups of Oats
- 1 Cup of Buckwheat
- 1 Cup of Sunflower Seeds
- 1 Cup of Pumpkin Seeds
- 1 ½ Cups of Dates, Pitted
- 1 Cup of Apple Puree
- 6 Tablespoons of Oil, Coconut Variety
- 4 Tablespoons of Cacao, Raw and Powdered Variety
- 1 Piece of Ginger

zzzzzzzzzzzzzzzzzzzzzzzzzzzzzzzzzzzzzzzzzzzzzzzzzzzzz

Instructions:

1. The first thing that you will want to do is preheat your oven to 350 degrees.

2. Then place your oats, buckwheat and seeds into a large sized mixing bowl and stir well to combine.

3. Then add in your dates, pumpkin and oil into your saucepan and allow them to cook over medium heat for the next 5 minutes or until your dates are soft to the touch.

4. Transfer your mixture into a food processor along with your cacao powder and blend until smooth in consistency. Pour this mixture into your buckwheat and oat mixture and stir well to combine.

5. The generously grease a large sized baking dish with some coconut oil and spread your granola into them.

6. Place into your oven to bake for the next 40 minutes or until crispy to the touch.

7. Remove and allow to cool completely before serving. Enjoy.

25) Lemon Salmon with Zucchini

This is a quick and easy dish that you can put together with ease. This salmon is packed full of so much flavor; I know you won't be able to get enough of it.

Serving Sizes: 4 Servings

Preparation Time: 35 Minutes

Ingredient List:

- 4 Zucchini, Finely Chopped
- 2 Tablespoons of Olive Oil, Extra Virgin Variety
- Dash of Salt and Pepper, For Taste

Ingredients for Your Salmon:

- 2 Tablespoons of Brown Sugar, Light and Packed
- 2 Tablespoons of Lemon Juice, Fresh
- 1 tablespoon of Mustard, Dijon Variety
- 2 Cloves of Garlic, Minced
- ½ teaspoons of Dill, Dried
- ½ teaspoons of Oregano, Dried Variety
- ¼ teaspoons of Thyme, Dried Variety
- ¼ teaspoons of Rosemary, Dried Variety
- Dash of Salt and Pepper, For Taste
- 4, 5 Ounce Fillets of Salmon
- 2 Tablespoons of Parsley Leaves, Fresh and Roughly Chopped

zzzzzzzzzzzzzzzzzzzzzzzzzzzzzzzzzzzzzzzzzzzzzzzzzzz

Instructions:

1. First preheat your oven to 400 Degrees. While your oven is heating up line a baking sheet with some cooking spray.

2. Then use a small sized bowl and mix together your first 10 ingredients for your salmon until thoroughly combined. Set this mixture aside.

3. Next place your zucchini into a single layer onto your baking sheet. Drizzle your olive oil over the top and season was some salt and pepper.

4. Then add your salmon in a single layer onto your baking sheet and brush each fillet with your herb mixture.

5. Place into your oven to bake for the next 16 to 18 minutes or until your fish is able to flake off easily with a fork.

6. After this time remove and serve with a garnish of parsley.

26) Sweet Potato and Roasted Red Pepper Soup

This is a great tasting delicious soup recipe to make if you are looking for a dish that is packed full of flavor. These two ingredients come together perfectly making a soup recipe you won't be able to resist.

Serving Sizes: 6 Servings

Preparation Time: 55 Minutes

Ingredient List:

- 2 Tablespoons of Olive Oil, Extra Virgin Variety
- 2 Onions, Medium in Size and Finely Chopped
- 1, 12 Ounce Jar of Red Peppers, Roasted Variety and Finely Chopped
- 1, 4 Ounce Can of Green Chiles, Finely Diced
- 2 teaspoons of Cumin, Ground Variety
- 1 teaspoon of Salt, For Taste
- 1 teaspoon of Coriander, Ground Variety
- 3 to 4 Cups of Sweet Potatoes, Peeled and Cut into Cubes
- 4 Cups of Broth, Vegetable Variety
- 2 Tablespoons of Cilantro, Fresh and Minced
- 1 tablespoon of Lemon Juice, Fresh
- 4 Ounces of Cream Cheese, Cut into Cubes

zzzzzzzzzzzzzzzzzzzzzzzzzzzzzzzzzzzzzzzzzzzzzzzzzzz

Instructions:

1. Using a large sized soup pot, heat up your olive oil over medium to high heat. Once the oil is hot enough add in your onions and cook until they are soft to the touch

2. Then add in your next 5 ingredients and continue to cook for an additional 1 to 2 minutes.

3. Add in your reserved juice for your roasted red peppers along with your next 2 ingredients. Bring your mixture to a boil before reducing the heat to low.

4. Cover and continue to cook until your potatoes are tender to the touch. This should take at least 10 to 15 minutes.

5. After this time add in your cilantro and lemon juice and stir to combine. Remove from heat and allow to cool slightly.

6. Pour in your soup into a blender along with your cream cheese. Blend on the highest setting until smooth in consistency. Pour this back into your pot and heat over low heat until hot to the touch.

7. Season with additional salt before serving. Enjoy.

About the Author

A native of Albuquerque, New Mexico, Sophia Freeman found her calling in the culinary arts when she enrolled at the Sante Fe School of Cooking. Freeman decided to take a year after graduation and travel around Europe, sampling the cuisine from small bistros and family owned restaurants from Italy to Portugal. Her bubbly personality and inquisitive nature made her popular with the locals in the villages and when she finished her trip and came home, she had made friends for life in the places she had visited. She also came home with a deeper understanding of European cuisine.

Freeman went to work at one of Albuquerque's 5-star restaurants as a sous-chef and soon worked her way up to head chef. The restaurant began to feature Freeman's original dishes as specials on the menu and soon after, she began to write e-books with her recipes. Sophia's dishes mix local flavours with European inspiration making them irresistible to the diners in her restaurant and the online community.

Freeman's experience in Europe didn't just teach her new ways of cooking, but also unique methods of presentation. Using rich sauces, crisp vegetables and meat cooked to perfection, she creates a stunning display as well as a delectable dish. She has won many local awards for her cuisine and she continues to delight her diners with her culinary masterpieces.

Author's Afterthoughts

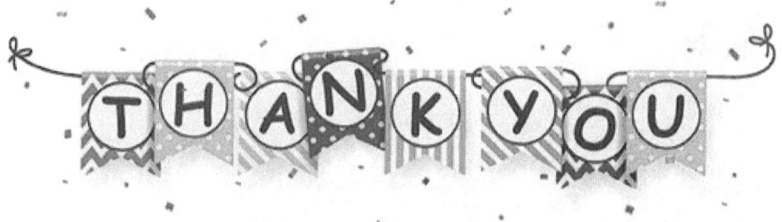

I want to convey my big thanks to all of my readers who have taken the time to read my book. Readers like you make my work so rewarding and I cherish each and every one of you.

Grateful cannot describe how I feel when I know that someone has chosen my work over all of the choices available online. I hope you enjoyed the book as much as I enjoyed writing it.

Feedback from my readers is how I grow and learn as a chef and an author. Please take the time to let me know your thoughts by leaving a review on Amazon so I and your fellow readers can learn from your experience.

My deepest thanks,

Sophia Freeman

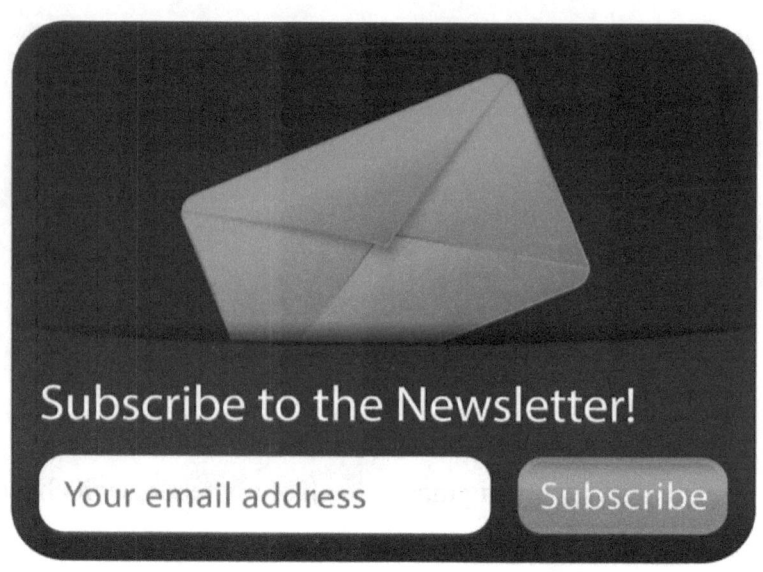

Subscribe to the Newsletter!

Your email address · Subscribe

https://sophia.subscribemenow.com/